Essential Oils For Allergies

The Complete Guide To Curing Allergies Using The Natural Power Of Essential Oils

By Amy Joyson

Disclaimer – Please read!

The information provided in this book is designed to provide helpful information on the subjects discussed. This book is not meant to be used, nor should it be used, to diagnose or treat any medical condition. For diagnosis or treatment of any medical problem, consult your own physician. The publisher and author are not responsible for any specific health or allergy needs that may require medical supervision and are not liable for any damages or negative consequences from any treatment, action, application or preparation, to any person reading or following the information in this book. References are provided for informational purposes only and do not constitute endorsement of any websites or other sources. Readers should be aware that the websites listed in this book may change.

Chapter 1- Introduction to Allergies............................6

Allergy Statistics—The Shocking Figures 6

Allergic Inflammatory Response............................7

Chapter 2- Aromatherapy and How it Can be Used to Improve Health............................9

Chapter 3- Practical Applications of Aromatherapy.15

Chapter 4- Cautions When Using Essential Oils........19

What age is safe to use what oils?............................21

Ages under 3 months 21

Ages 3+ months 21

Ages 6+ months 22

Ages 2+ years............................22

Ages 6+ years............................23

Ages 10+ years............................24

Chapter 5- Blending Essential Oils for Powerful Allergy Fighters............................25

Condition 25

Essential Oil............................25

Application 25

Chapter 6- Using Essential Oils Every Day............................28

Chapter 7- Conclusion............................30

2 FREE eBooks for you!............................ 32

About The Author............................34

Valerian Press............................35

Preview Of My Book "Essential Oil Massage Techniques For Beginners"............................ 36

Chapter 1- Introduction to Allergies

A popular and ever growing trend today is the use of essential oils to treat a wide range of health issues. They are not just for health nuts and hippies and more and more people are discovering the great benefits essential oils offer. One of the popular treatments that use these natural oils is for seasonal allergies, one of the most common conditions that cause people suffering from allergies to first look to essential oils.

Allergy Statistics—The Shocking Figures

In the US every year it is estimated that about 24 million adults and children are diagnosed with some sort of seasonal allergies. The American Allergy Foundation of America (AAFA) has some staggering figures that cannot be ignored: "Allergy is the 5th leading chronic disease in the U.S. among all ages, and the 3rd most common chronic disease among children under 18 years old. Each year, allergies account for more than 17 million outpatient office visits, primarily in the spring and fall; seasonal allergies account for more than half of all allergy visits. For adults, allergies (hay fever) is the 5th leading chronic disease and a major cause of work absenteeism." With numbers like that, which only seem to grow with each passing year, a logical question is what is the cost of such widespread allergy suffering?

On a whole, Americans spend $14.5 billion on allergy medication, treatment, doctor's visits, and missed work/school each year. Seasonal allergies are thought to count for half of these instances with food allergies making up the other half. Despite new advances in medicine and new allergy drugs coming out every few years, things are not improving. Allergy prevalence continues to rise as pollen counts soar and allergy season spans continue to grow longer each and every year. Changes in climate, increased pollution, plant and landscape choices, overall health standards, and other factors are all helping to contribute to more severe cases of allergies across the country.

Allergic Inflammatory Response

The body is designed to help protect itself from the impact of allergy inducing triggers, known as allergens. Our eyes, nose, and skin do a great job of keeping outside contaminants out of the body. However, when allergens get past these first lines of defense, the immune system steps in and goes to work. In people who are "allergic," these normally benign allergens are mistakenly seen by the immune system as a threat, which will cause the white blood cells to release histamine as a step to rid the body of the invaders and to protect against further invasion. This leads to the typical allergic reactions allergy sufferers are all too familiar with. "Allergy is characterized by an overreaction of the human immune system to a foreign protein substance ("allergen") that is eaten, breathed into the lungs, injected or touched. This immune overreaction can result in symptoms such as coughing, sneezing, itchy eyes, runny nose and scratchy throat. In severe cases it can also result in rashes, hives, lower blood pressure, difficulty breathing, asthma attacks, and even death" (AAFA).

For most people these symptoms are very uncomfortable and for many, they are completely debilitating. People with major seasonal allergies to things such as pollen, dust, and animal dander can even experience serious reactions including difficulty breathing and hives. These severe reactions are the body's attempt to remove the allergen from the body- by sneezing and flushing it out.

Many people are under the false assumption that an over-reactive immune system that produce these sorts of reactions to simple triggers means that it is too strong. A hyperactive immune system is not *too strong*. What is happening is that the immune system is *misfiring and suffering from over reaction*, which is a sign of weakness. An immune system that is healthy and strong is discerning and can better distinguish a real threat from the imaginary ones that often cause severe seasonal allergies. It targets real threats like bacteria, viruses, and parasites, and will ignore harmless pollens. This is how a healthy immune system works and how things should be when things are functioning properly. When the body's natural defenses fail and misfire, people look for ways to alleviate the symptoms; most people turn to medications and expensive pharmaceutical drugs. For a natural and safer option, essential oils are gaining more attention and are becoming more popular every year.

Chapter 2- Aromatherapy and How it Can be Used to Improve Health

Aromatherapy is the practice of using essential oils to naturally treat various medical disorders and conditions ranging from the common cold to arthritis to indigestion. Essential oils are made from infusing and distilling liquids that have been taken from plants. They can be wonderfully fragrant and many have great benefits that they can bring with extended use. You have experienced the benefits of aromatic essential oils if you enjoy the smell of freshly cut oranges, the scent of lavender blooms, felt better after smelling warm vanilla scents, or felt yourself relax after smelling sea salt. Essential oils are super-concentrated. For example, it takes about 16 pounds of fresh peppermint leaves to produce an ounce of essential oil. These oils constitute important active ingredients and flavor additives in many kinds of familiar, everyday products — candies, syrups, toothpastes, mouthwashes, cleaning products, skin creams, lip balms, shampoos, bath salts, and soaps. Essential oils even give flavor and aroma to the spices that you use to add zest to your cooking, such as cinnamon, allspice, and nutmeg used for apple cider, pies, and baked goods. Nutmeg, allspice, thyme, oregano, basil, and savory all contain essential oils.

Smells can do amazing things and trigger memories, feelings, and physical changes we may not even be aware of at that moment and time. Essential oils are more than just an alternative to perfume or air fresheners. They have been used in all of mankind's history for centuries thanks to their natural healing properties. With the growth in trends that look towards a more holistic approach to wellness, more and more people are discovering the benefits of essential oils and are using them in their day to day life and enjoying the benefits. A study conducted in 2004 at the Department of Organic and Bioorganic Chemistry at Lund University in Sweden showed the effectiveness of a Nasal Spray formulated with the essential oils of Eucalyptus (cineole), Lavender (linalool) and Cypress (davanone). After administration of the nasal spray, all patients experienced a rapid and significant relief of nasal symptoms, comparable to the effect of antihistamine. The effect was present within 5 minutes after the administration and lasted for several hours. This is just one example of how essential oils are being used and formulated for easy use and further exemplifies the attraction people have for these natural remedies.

Turn to aromatherapy as a natural alternative instead of using an over-the-counter drug to ease a cold, headache, indigestion, or bee sting — the simple complaints that you already take care of yourself without consulting your doctor. After all, that's what aroma*therapy* is — a healing therapy. The *aroma* part of the word refers is to the aromatic plants that are used in this therapy. Here are some of the common essential oils that people have found helpful in dealing with the symptoms of allergy flare ups:

Eucalyptus – one of the most popular oils, this fragrant oil helps to fight symptoms including congestion, headaches, and respiratory conditions. There is also powerful instances of anti-inflammatory, disinfectant, and expectorant properties, which is why eucalyptus is commonly used in muscle rub and cough drops. When mixed with a carrier oil topical application to chest and throat is also helpful and helps speed relief of even the worst symptoms.

Peppermint – aids breathing and reduces the constriction of the chest and throat by opening sinuses and airways. It is also helpful in fighting infection, relieving the pain of headache and muscular strains, and it also has powerful anti-inflammatory properties. Carrier mixes can be use on the temples, neck, and chest to send powerful relief quickly and reduce the severity and duration of symptoms.

Lemon – the essential oil blend of lemon boosts immunity, improves blood flow, and relieves respiratory issues. It is an excellent antibacterial agent, making it a great allergy fighting component for many aroma therapy uses. Lemon essential oil helps clean the environment and the air, which helps remove allergens from the air and makes them less likely to trigger allergic reactions in the first place.

Lavender – perhaps the most commonly used essential oil, lavender is known to have powerful anti-inflammatory properties, to be important to building and strengthening immunity, helping in relieving headaches and muscle pain, and it also is powerful as a natural antihistamine. It has a very calming and relaxing, soothing aroma that many people find enjoyable and comforting, which makes it great for use every day and in a variety of essential oil blends.

Roman Chamomile – a newer blend for the essential oils, this offering has great anti-inflammatory, relaxing, and pain relieving properties. As a powerful antispasmodic and muscle relaxant some people have found it helpful for allergy relief to indoor stimulants such as dust and mold but not as useful for outdoor allergies such as pollen.

Cypress – antispasmodic and disinfectant, this essential oil is used in aroma therapy for a range of applications, but it is very beneficial when used on its own or in blends to help with allergy symptoms. It helps to relieve breathing difficulties and suppress coughing while helping to make the cough that remains more productive.

Ginger – as an analgesic, expectorant and stimulant, ginger has a great smell that many people enjoy. It has been shown to help decreases respiratory symptoms including constricted airways, wheezing, nasal and chest congestion, and coughing. Many people like the smell of ginger so it is a great oil that can be used in a number of ways to help deal with allergy symptoms.

"Essential oils can help balance and support the body to heal itself. Research has shown that essential oils help us fight infection, contain balancing compounds and aid regeneration. They possess anti-bacterial, anti-fungal and anti-viral properties" (Heritage Essential Oils). One way to achieve the maximum help and benefit from the essential oils that you decide to use is to massage the carrier and oil mix around the neck and behind the ears. Another way to get treatment throughout the day is to have a handkerchief that you add a few drops of the oil to and inhale it deeply a few times throughout the day as needed for on the go relief. To fight severe congestion, especially night time pressure before bed, add a few drops of your chosen oils in a bowl with hot steaming water. Drape a towel over your head and lean over the bowl and breathe in the vapors.

To relieve severe or persistent allergy symptoms combine two drops of your essential oils in a small amount of water. You can take the mix and use it as a gargle and mouth rinse to get some relief from the sinus symptoms and pain. Diffuse the oils in a room with a special steam or wick diffuser to give all day and all night relief from your allergy symptoms. For bed time relief of your allergy symptoms, add a few drops of oil to your pillow. One of the best ways to get the best result from your essential oils is to use them a month before your allergy season starts and to continue using them for a month after to ensure you stay as healthy as possible. However you choose to use oils there are many ways they can help speed comfort to even your worst allergy symptoms.

Here are some important facts that can help you get the best use out of your essential oils:
To test and see if your essential oil is as "pure" as someone has told you it is, put a single drop of it onto some construction paper. If it evaporates quickly and there is a lack of a noticeable ring, then it is safe to say that it is pretty pure. If you have a ring left, then the manufacturer has likely already diluted it with an oil. You do not want this because you dilute the oils on your own before using them and you want the strong concentration of oils since that is what you are paying for. Note, this test will not work for some oils such as myrrh,

patchouli, and absolutes due to their composition.

Essential oils have been used since ancient times and one reason for its long lasting popularity is that pure essential oils will last for at least 5 years or even 10 years or more! They may cost a lot, but one bottle can last a decade because so little is needed for medicinal purposes. The only real exception to this rule of longevity is citrus oils, which tends to start to break down and lose its potency after a 2 or 3 years.

To test for possible sensitivity to a particular essential oil, which is best done before using it for skin care or in diffusers, follow this simple test. Combine one drop of your chosen type of essential oil with 1/2 tsp carrier oil -olive, jojoba, grapeseed, and coconut being popular options. Rub this mixture on the inside, upper area of the arm and wait a few hours. If there has been no reaction, no redness, and no itching then you are most likely not sensitive to that oil and can begin the gradual addition and increase in concentration until you reach the level that is best for you.

Essential oils are seen as a completely natural product and as such they cannot be patented; this means that essential oils will not be used in a pharmaceutical drug. Because of this, most mainstream healthcare practitioners do not openly recommend essential oils to their patients and they are not fond of recommending them as therapeutic alternatives to drugs- only homeopathic practitioners openly embrace essential oils for medicinal treatments.

Since essential oils cannot be patented, they are of little use to mainstream drug companies and as such they will not spend the time or money necessary to fully study them and learn about their use, benefits, and applications. This limits scientific knowledge of essential oils by a great deal, and the majority of what is known about the benefits and use of essential oils have been passed down through thousands of years of records, trials, experiments, studies, and personal usage.

Chapter 3- Practical Applications of Aromatherapy

As already discussed, aromatherapy is the act of using fragrances and aromas to distress, ease pain, relieve tension, and health spirit, mind, and body. There are many fragrances that are used and there are many different ailments that can be helped through aromatherapy and the use of essential oils and blends. So, how do you use essential oils?

There are three basic ways to enjoy the maximum benefits of the therapeutic essential oils:

Aromatically – This refers to the simple act of inhaling steam that has been infused with an essential oil. This is a popular method as it can bring immediate results to begin relieving even the worst allergy symptoms. Diffusing essentials oils helps clean the air and will rid the air of unwanted odors and also goes a long way to purify the air and remove pathogens.

Topically – Essential oils are a natural product and are easily absorbed through the skin, making them easy to apply topically when done correctly. Essential oils are very concentrated and potent so they should be mixed with a carrier oil before they are applied to the skin in order to avoid irritating the skin. With essential oils, less is always more, and it is important to remember that only a few drops are needed to achieve the desired results.

Internally –This is the least common method of essential oil use as it is the most risky due to the highly concentrated nature of the oils. Some essential oils work as dietary supplements to help with allergy symptoms and other common issues and ailments. Many essential oils are generally recognized as safe, but there are also some that should never be ingested so it is important to check with an authority site or someone knowledgeable in essential oils before you take any essential oil by mouth.

When considering the quality of essential oil, you always want to make sure you get an oil that is guaranteed to be 100% pure and natural and free of synthetic compounds or contaminates. That being said, even though the label may say 100% pure, it is not always the case. Do your homework, and really look into the company that is marketing the essential oil. What kind of independent testing do they do to make sure their oils are pure? Where do they source their oils? Also keep in mind that higher quality therapeutic grade oil is going to cost a bit more than perfume quality oil

Additionally, there are many places in your daily life that can utilize aromatherapy:

Bathroom
Shower oils, soaps, bath salts, and fragrance infused shower systems are becoming very popular throughout the United States. The abundance of steam makes them a great place to utilize the benefits of essential oils and the benefits of warm steam. If the cost of special aroma therapy shower system is not feasible, an alternative method is to drop some oil on the washcloth, sponge, or poof and generate aroma filled suds to enjoy.

Kitchen
While you often want to smell the fragrance of what you are cooking, certain tasks done in the kitchen are not very fun and having some nicely scented candles burning or some incense can help make those tasks more enjoyable. Oil burners and diffusers can help you deal with that allergy flare up after taking out the garbage or to help minimize the sinus flare up after doing yard work.

Living   *room*
Visit with friends and family and keep the atmosphere calm and relaxed with a nice essential oil fragrance and make it

easier to enjoy the company without the drama and stress of a big get together. Many essential oils offer a pleasing aroma that everyone will love.

Bedroom
Millions of Americans struggle to sleep well at night because of allergy symptoms and sinus related issues. A simple act like burning some essential oil candles, taking an essential oil steam bath, or using another aromatherapy session before bed can go a long way in helping the mind and body relax and prepare for sleep. Infusing your pillows or mattress with a little oil blend can also offer all night aromatherapy to help make sleep easier and deeper.

Garage
The garage is usually not the best smelling place to be nor is it the most relaxing place to be when work needs to be done, but that is quickly changed when you add in some refreshing and energizing aromas to the mix. Keep the allergens at bay and keep the air clean with aromatherapy.

Car
Few people think about using aromatherapy in the car but when you consider the fact that nowadays people spend almost a third of their lives in their vehicles, it make sense to consider this as a viable aromatherapy place.

Office
The average worker can spend almost half his or her life at work, and everyone know the stress that work can bring, and some aromatherapy ideas can work well for the office of cubicle and can make that desk job less stressful. Small desk diffusers or oil dripped tissues can offer a discrete yet powerful source of relief throughout the day.

If you decide to get more personal with your essential oils and use them directly on your skin as topical applications, then you need to ensure that you are only using pure high quality grade therapeutic oils. There are several elements that are necessary for the production of high quality oils that can be considered therapeutic essential oil. First, there needs to be a good plant grown in healthy soil according to organic growing methods. Second, the plants must be patiently distilled by means of the best steam distillation procedures. Third, the purity of the extracted oil must be maintained by avoiding the use of solvents and assuring its quality by analysis with gas chromatography and a mass spectrometer. It's only by carefully producing therapeutic oils in this way that they can promote health and well-being. This is because it's only through this process that all the vital constituent parts of the therapeutic oil can be secured.

Chapter 4- Cautions When Using Essential Oils

Everything in moderation, essential oils included. They can be a wonderful way to treat allergy symptoms naturally, but they are potent so it is important to do your research before you start using them, buy high-grade oils, and always be sure you use them wisely. Be especially cautious if essential oils are being used around children as some of them are not intended for little ones.

Although essential oils can be beneficial they are still a form of medication and must be treated with the same respect prescription medications are given. Taking too much of an essential oil in too high a concentration can cause serious side effects in some people, which is why they must always be diluted in oil blends and diluted in water if taken orally or applied directly to the skin.

When buying essential oils check the containers to ensure the seals are still intact and that the droppers and lids are still attached. Make sure labels are included and that there is a dosage guide as well as a proof of concentration and purity printed on the labels. Never buy damaged bottles of bottles that have missing labels.

Keep all essential oils in an out of reach safe place – small children should not be able to get a hold of them, and a cool dark place will slows the oxidation of the oils and helps them keep their potency for longer.

Never use essential oils undiluted on the skin, and if using them on children under the age of 12, remember to use a dilution of at least half strength. For children under the age of 6, many experts recommend using a quarter strength concentration.

Many different oils can be used as a carrier oil to dilute the oil blends. Common oils include grapeseed oil, olive oil, sunflower oil, safflower oil, vegetable oil, or coconut oil.

Limit exposure to steam and air diffusers and never allow young children to use essential oils unsupervised.

Remember that dilution is very important for all essential oils, no exceptions! No matter what essential oil you sue, the brand, or how you are using it, no essential oil is safe in its concentrate form. It is also important to note that when adding essential oils to baths of children, they must first be diluted in a water soluble carrier, such as raw unfiltered honey or vegetable glycerin. Adding essential oils straight to bath water, without a carrier, runs you the risk of causing irritation to the skin. There are many applications for essential oils with babies and children, but they should be kept away from a child's face. To ensure safety when using essential oils, rubbing the diluted oils on the soles of the feet is often the safest way to apply the oil to young children and many adults find the best benefits from applying oils to the feet as well.

Slowly introduce one essential oil at a time to avoid reactions and sudden shock due to too much exposure too quickly. Remember that every essential oil is different so just because you or your family are fine with one does not mean that they will be fine with another oil. So every new oil needs to be slowly introduced over a period of a week or two before adding in any other oils. It's important to introduce every essential oils one at a time and as sparingly as possible as you slowly build to the target amount. If a blend calls for lemon, eucalyptus, and ginger oils, start with one and use it at a quarter strength for a few days and then build until that oil is at full strength and you go 3-5 days with no adverse reaction. Then add the next oil in a quarter strength and replete the process. This is the best way to test out new oils and mixtures as it gives you a way to both watch for any sort of reaction and it lets the body naturally adjust and absorb the oils. Use these oils as directed... and do it morning and night for at least a week before you jump to any conclusions. And if it doesn't work, or it doesn't work as well as you'd like, it might be your body chemistry is slightly different and will respond better to a different combination of oils. There's some trial and error involved at times, so proceed with some caution and start small, then work from there. In most cases a reaction to essential oils are fairly quick and adverse reaction after inhalation or dermal application are usually visible in as little as 15 minutes and usually will manifest within 2 hours.

What age is safe to use what oils?

This is a question that many people wonder, whether they are using the essential oils directly on their children or not. There is a lot of good information to be found on essential oils if you do your research, but there is still very little known in regards to the safety of essential oils when it comes to use with babies and children. It is often suggested to use your judgment and to consult with a doctor or homeopathic expert when it comes to choosing essential oils to use in your home -whether for yourself or for your family.

Ages under 3 months

Essential oils are not recommended to be used with babies less than 3 months of age because they are not mature enough and their skin, lungs, and bodies are not properly prepared to deal with the addition of essential oils into their system. It is widely recommended that essential oils are never used before the age of 3 months old and even then they should only be used with extreme care and only under the advice and guidance of a pediatrician or trained expert. There are no widely accepted oils that are safe for infants younger than 6 months of age.

Ages 3+ months

The maximum advisable amount of essential oils for infants of at least 3 months of age should not exceed .2% of the recipe, or

1-2 drops of essential oil per ounce of carrier oil. Following are the essential oils that are thought to be safe for infants:

- Chamomile, Roman and German (*Anthemis nobilis, Matricaria rectutita*)
- Dill (*Anthum graveolens*)
- Lavender – (*Lavendula angustifolia*)
- Yarrow, Blue (*Achillea millefolium*)

Ages 6+ months

Even at 6 months old, many infants are too immature to properly handle essential oils and many experts advise that they not be used unless as a last effort to treat certain conditions or if supervised by a pediatrician. Essential oils used with babies 6+ months must not exceed the level of .5% of the recipe, or 3-5 drops of essential oil per ounce of carrier oil. Here are some of the common essential oils that are thought to be safe for this age group and that are useful for treating common childhood illnesses and conditions:

- Bergamot (*Citrus bergamia*)
- Carrot Seed (*Daucus carota*)
- Citronella (*Cymbopogon nardus*)
- Cypress (*Cupressus sempervires*)
- Geranium (*Pelargonium graveolens*)
- Grapefruit (*Citrus paradisi*)
- Lemon (*Citrus limon*)
- Mandarin (*Citrus reticulata*)
- Pine (*pinus*)
- Ravensara (*Ravensara aromatica*)
- Rose Otto (*Rosa damascena*)
- Sandalwood (*Santalum spicatum*)
- Spruce (*picea*)
- Sweet Orange (*Citrus sinensis*)
- Tea Tree (*Melaleuca alternifolia*)

Ages 2+ years

Once a child has reached the age of 2, it is safer and easier to use essential oils in diffusions as well as topical application, but care but still be taken. The maximum recommended quantity for essential oils in this age group is no more than 2% of the recipe, or 20 drops of essential oil per ounce of carrier oil. Following are the common essential oils that become safer to use at this age, in addition to the ones previously mentioned:

- Basil, Lemon (*Ociumum x citriodorum*)
- Basil, Sweet (*Ocimum basilicum*)
- Benzoin (*Styrax benzoin*)
- Clary Sage (*Salvia sclarea*)
- Frankincense (*Boswellia carterii*)
- Garlic (*Allium sativum*)
- Ginger (*Zingiber officinale*)
- Hyssop (*Hyssopus officinalis*)
- Juniper Berry (*Juniperus communis*)
- Lemongrass (*Andropogon citratus*)
- Lime (*Cirtus x aurantifolia*)
- Myrrh (*Commiphora myrrha*)
- Oregano (*Origanum*)
- Sweet Marjoram (*Marjorana hortensis*)
- Patchouli (*Pogostemon* cablin)
- Spearmint (*Mentha cardiaca, Mentha spicata*)
- Tea Tree, Lemon (*Leptospermum*)
- Thyme (*Thymus vulgaris, Thymus Zygis*)
- Tumeric (*Cucuma longa*)
- Valarian (*Valeriana officinalis*)
- Ylang Ylang (*Cananga odorata*)

Ages 6+ years

When working with essential oils at any age, great care should be taken and you must be sure to research each essential oil's warnings, guidelines, and concentration before using. The highest strength of oils that can be used on children 6+ years should be no higher than 3% of the recipe, or 30 drops of essential oil per ounce of carrier oil. At this age, there are many common conditions that essential oils can treat, such as colds, upset stomach, sleeplessness, irritability, and many others. Following are some of the additional oils that are thought to be safe for this age group:

- Anise/Aniseed (*Pimpinella anisum)*
- Anise, Star (I*llicium verum*)
- Cajuput (*Melaleuca cajuputi, Melaleuca leucadendron*)
- Cardamom (*Elettaria cardamomum*)
- Cornmint (*Mentha arvensis, Mentha canadensis*)
- Fennel (*Foeniculum vulgare*)
- Laurel Leaf/Bay Laurel (*Laurus nobilis*)
- Marjoram (*Thymus mastichina*)
- Niaouli (*cineole chemotype*)
- Nutmeg (*Myristica fragrans*)
- Sage, Greek/White (*Salvia*)

Ages 10+ years

By this age, it is considered safe to use most essential oils for topical application or for diffusion; however, you should always make sure you follow the cautions given already and slowly introduce new oils and keep the concentrations low and build slowly. Keep a close eye on your children and watch for any adverse reactions or problems while using the oils. Peppermint, eucalyptus, and rosemary essential oils are all avoided in younger children because they contain a chemical constituent called cineol 1,8 and menthol. According to Robert Tisserand, in the newest edition of Essential Oil Safety: This is the reason that it is suggested to avoid the use of these essential oils (and others containing a high content of these chemical constituents) in young children. Peppermint is safe to use at 6+ years but ALL eucalyptus and rosemary essential oils should be avoided until 10+ years of age. It's important to note that the brand of essential oil you choose to use does not change this recommendation."

Chapter 5- Blending Essential Oils for Powerful Allergy Fighters

Many people live on anti-histamines and decongestants or prescription medication through allergy season. Others choose to receive allergy shots several times during the year for relief. However, many people are now looking for a more natural solution. One option that can help allergy symptoms is Aromatherapy. In fact, they offer a great alternative for allergy sufferers.

Following are some of the common allergy and relating symptoms along with the essential oils that are effective against them as well as the recommended methods of application.

Condition	Essential Oil	Application
Acne, Rash, Hives- Other Allergic Reactions	Tea Tree, Lavender	Topical When Diluted
Allergies and related congestion and dripping	Wintergreen, Lavender, Chamomile	Steam Inhalation, Topical- Recommended on Feet
Apnea and Other Sleep Issues Related to Repository Conditions	Blends of Lavender, Wintergreen, and Chamomile	Inhalation Through Steam, Topical- Chest and Feet When Diluted
Asthma	Wintergreen, Eucalyptus, Lavender, Frankincense, Lemon	Use Topically on Feet and Chest Only When Diluted

Blisters and Rash	German Chamomile, Tea Tree, Melrose, Lavender	Topical on Site When Diluted
Blocked Tear Duct - Nasal Congestion or Sinus Infection	Lavender, Eucalyptus	Topically Applied to Nose When Diluted Properly
Bronchitis	Myrtle, Pine, Eucalyptus, Balsam Fir	Topical at Diluted Strength, Steam Inhalation
Colds	Eucalyptus, Peppermint, Lemon	Topical Application to Nose and Chest When Diluted, Steam Inhalation, and Supervised Ingestion
Cough	Peppermint, Eucalyptus	Inhalation of Steam, Topical Use of Diluted Oils on Chest and Throat
Dizziness	Peppermint, Frankincense, Cedarwood	Inhalation, Topical
Earache From Congestion/Infection	Wintergreen, Melrose, Eucalyptus	Topical on Head Around Ears- Never in the Ears Directly
Headache From Sinus Congestion and Allergy Flares	Peppermint, Wintergreen, Lemon, Vanilla	Steam Inhalation, Dilution of Topical Application, Oral Ingestion by Gargling
Insect Bites and Related Allergic Reactions-Mild	Peppermint, Melrose, Citronella, Lavender, Tea tree	Topical Application of Diluted Oils to Bite
Sinus Congestion	Eucalyptus,	Inhalation of

	Peppermint	Steam, Topical Use of Properly Diluted Oils
Stress	Lavender, Frankincense, Vanilla	Inhalation of Steam, Topical Application of Diluted Blends

A word of caution when you begin blending and using essential oils for your allergy relief: Only choose quality oils! There are a multitude of companies that intentionally mislead customers by making claims that they offer "pure", "therapeutic grade" or "aromatherapy grade" essential oils. It is important to know that as of yet, there are no government regulations concerning the production and sale of essential oils and no government body has control over how companies label or certify their essential oils.

You can, however, find high quality organic essential oils and ones that are perfectly safe to use; all you have to do is a little research when shopping and make sure you do not just buy the first essential oils you find online. When looking for quality oils, make sure that all of the following are clearly visible on the original labeling:

Common or brand name of essential oil (i.e. Lavender)
Latin name of essential oil (i.e. Lavendula angustifolia)
Country of origin (i.e. USA)
How oil was extracted (i.e. steam distilled)

By taking the time to do your research before you buy and start blending your own essential oils, you can ensure that you and your family are getting the best quality oils and that you can stay as happy and healthy and safe as you possibly can!

Chapter 6- Using Essential Oils Every Day

No bath or body product would be complete without an enticing scent! Our sense of smell is intricately tied to our memories and emotions, so the right aroma is key; it can transport you to a lush forest or bring to mind the zingy scent of your favorite fruit....concentrated essential oils are perfect for adding scent to lotions, massage oils, body butters, perfumes, or soaps. Use eucalyptus oils to help soothe aches and relieve tight muscles, add some vanilla and lavender oils to your bath to soak away the stress and anxiety, or use natural soaps that use revitalizing and cleaning oils that help clear the sinuses- lemongrass, ginger, cedar and frankincense.

One great way to use essential oils with the maximum efficiency is to find soaps, bath salts, lotions, and other bath and beauty products that have essential oils in them. Unlike store-bought soaps that are made with a lot of harsh chemicals, all-natural soap products are safe for your body and when they are made with essential oils, you can get the benefits of the oil in an easy to use safe dose each and every day. Natural soaps smell fresh and have a cleansing, skin-smoothing effect. The vast majority of handmade soaps use natural oils as the key ingredients and also use essential oils for the fragrance, natural healing, and revitalizing effects. Handmade soaps utilize therapeutic essential oils and this makes it easy to find a soap that can help with your allergy relief.

Soaps made with the essential oils that help relieve congestion, soothe the sinuses, clear stuffiness, and helps clear the body of irritating histamines are a great way to have a a personal allergy treatment session right in your shower, anytime you have a need. Many people do not fully realize the health benefits that come from washing with pure all natural soaps that use essential oils for allergy relief. So look for soaps that list natural oils and have a listing of essential oils on the ingredient labels and enjoy an aromatherapy session today that utilizes the effects of vanilla, eucalyptus, citrus, lemongrass, cedar, lavender, frankincense, peppermint, chamomile, and many, many more!

Chapter 7- Conclusion

As we conclude our study of essential oils and how beneficial they can be to treat and relieve and even to help prevent common seasonal allergies, we conclude with the following ten things you need to remember about essential oils:

Essential oils have been used by cultures throughout the world for centuries. There are mentions of essential oils in the Bible and other ancient texts and writings and records of ancient cultures like the Indian and Chinese regions show that they have used plant based oils for a range of treatments.

Many essential oils offer amazing beneficial properties that are easy to enjoy with proper use. Oils can help boost the immune system, lift moods, clear skin, soothe soreness, and many other great uses. Essential oils contain powerful antioxidants that can help people have healthier, happier, and longer lives.

There are many ways to enjoy and use essential oils. Whether you use the oils as a topical application, in a diffuser, or taken orally you get great benefits. There are other fun and easy ways to use oils such as in your bath, in soaps and bath salts, lotions and oils, and many other creative ways.

They are absorbed easily by skin which is why so little oil needs to be used in a single application and why the oils need to be diluted in water or oils before being used. This quick and easy absorption allows for quick relief and long lasting results as he healing properties of the oils get into the bloodstream quickly and stay there.

Essential oils take a lot of plan material to make which is why they can be a bit pricey. A few drops of peppermint essential oil is the equivalent to almost 30 cups of peppermint tea. It takes a staggering 5,000 pounds of rose petals to make one pound of rose essential oil, making it among the most expensive oils on the market. Despite the work involved and the cost of some oils, we need to use such a small amount of essential oils that they last a long time and are still very economical.

Purity is absolutely critical! Do not try to cut costs by buying oils that are not pure and you have to take the time to do your research and investigate the oils and the companies you are looking to buy from. Essential oils can help you and your family be healthier but you have to ensure you are getting safe, high quality oils to start with.

Enjoy essential oils and discover a happier and healthier life for you and your family.

2 FREE eBooks for you!

Guys, thanks so much for reading my book. I truly hope it served as a great introduction to lavender essential oil. As a token of appreciation I have prepared two free ebooks for you. Here is a bit of information about them!

The 10 Most Important Essential Oils

In this book we delve deep into the uses and applications of the ten essential oils that I consider to be the most 'essential'. For each oil I explain the key health benefits, teach you the therapeutic applications and provide specific safety precaution. I include one of my most useful remedies for each of the oils as well. So you will receive a deep knowledge of ten essential oils and ten brilliant remedies for free! It is a 10k word eBook, the same length as this one!

When you receive this ebook you will also receive a couple of emails from me a week containing even more information about the essential oils! I will endeavour to give you at least 5 recipes or remedies per week and also provide you with some great information on the lesser known essential oils.

Simply click here to receive the ebooks!
Or type this link into a web browser: http://bit.ly/1EuHgyn

The Ultimate Guide To Vitamins

This is another wonderful 10k word ebook that has been made available to you through my publisher, Valerian Press. As a health conscious person you should be well aware of the uses and health benefits of each of the vitamins that should make up our diet. This book gives you an easy to understand, scientific explanation of the vitamin followed by the recommended daily dosage. It then highlights all the important health benefits of each vitamin. A list of the best sources of each vitamin is provided and you are also given some actionable next steps for each vitamin to make sure you are utilizing the information!

As well as receiving the free ebooks you will also be sent a weekly stream of free ebooks, again from my publishing company Valerian Press. You can expect to receive at least a new, free ebook each and every week. Sometimes you might receive a massive 10 free books in a week!

Simply click here to receive the ebooks!
Or type this link into a web browser: http://bit.ly/1EuHgyn

About The Author

Hey there! I'm Amy Joyson, a lifelong student of holistic and alternative medicine. My journey began as far back as I can remember, my mother, a practicing aromatherapist, taught me value of natural remedies as a youngster. I don't think I could imagine a life without the essential oils if I tried, they are just so important to me. I am passionate about sharing their value with as many people as possible, which led me to writing my books. If you have read any of my books I truly hope they have added value to your life and I thank you with all my heart for trusting in me.

Outside of being an author, I work as a personal trainer. Employing my deep knowledge of alternative treatments has enabled me to provide outstanding results for all of my clients!

In my spare time you will often find me lounging in my hammock reading the latest aromatherapy magazine or romantic fiction novel. I have a soft spot for true romance! I aim to meditate at least once a day, and practice yoga 5 times a week. My biggest hobby however is exploring the beautiful world that we live in. Next on my hit list is Iceland, there is something seriously alluring about that island.

You can find me here on Facebook: https://www.facebook.com/pages/Amy-Joyson/435155886642915

You can find me here on Twitter: https://twitter.com/Amy_Joyson

Valerian Press

At Valerian Press we have three key beliefs.

Providing outstanding value: We believe in enriching all of our customers' lives, doing everything we can to ensure the best experience.

Championing new talent: We believe in showcasing the worlds emerging talent by giving them the platform to grow.

Simplicity and efficiency: We understand how valuable your time is. Our products are stream-lined and consist only of what you want. You will find no fluff with us.

We hope you have enjoyed reading Amy's guide to curing allergies.

We would love to offer you a regular supply of our free and discounted books. We cover a huge range of non-fiction genres; diet and cookbooks, health and fitness, alternative and holistic medicine, spirituality and plenty more.

All you need to do is simply click here!
Alternatively you can type this link into your web browser: http://bit.ly/18hmup4

Preview Of My Book "Essential Oil Massage Techniques For Beginners"

Chapter 4 –Stress relief

Stress is one of the most debilitating and prolific health risks in society today. There is a proven and commonly accepted link between stress and poor health, yet many of us accept stress as just a part of our everyday lives. Our fast paced, high stakes, 'always on' world means that there is little (if any!) down time in many people's day-to-day schedules. Sadly, it is not an uncommon experience to feel as though you are holding on by your fingernails as life whips around you, while telling yourself that the one or two weeks of holiday planned in the distant future will be enough to keep you sane for another year. Fortunately, even though we may not be able to do a lot to change the things causing stress in our lives, we can take some steps to minimize the natural stress response of our bodies. There is perhaps no better way to calm one's nerves and elevated stress levels, than with a long, relaxing massage. As mentioned above, human touch can be highly effective in making us feel calm, a fact which is made possible through the hormonal chemistry of the human body. Prolonged touch between two people has been shown stimulate the release of the bonding chemical, oxytocin. This hormone is released in high doses through events in which human contact typically occurs, including hugging, kissing, sex and even light touch between two people. Most interestingly, at least when it comes to controlling our stress levels, oxytocin has been shown to have a *suppressant* effect on the body's stress hormone, cortisol. So that means that the more we expose ourselves to physical interactions with other people, the less cortisol induced stress we are likely to feel. When the stress relieving properties of certain essential oils are added into the mix, massage can provide a much needed reprieve for even the most cortisol stricken individuals. We'll now take a look at some of the most effective oils, blends and treatments for stress relief through the combination of aromatherapy and massage.

One of the best essential oils for inducing feelings of calm is lavender. Lavender is great for a whole range of therapeutic conditions – in fact, it is an absolutely *essential* essential oil. There are lots of essential oils that have loads of excellent and varied remedial properties, however, lavender is really queen when it comes to the world of aromatherapy. It is wonderfully versatile and can be applied for a range of purposes: from disinfecting wounds, to burns treatment, to pain relief. It is also one of the very few essential oils that can safely be applied to the skin 'neat' or undiluted. In summary, if you had to choose a 'desert island' essential oil, lavender should naturally be the go to option! Not least among the valued properties of lavender, is its ability to be utilized as an effective treatment for stress relief. Thanks to the versatility of lavender, we'll talk more about this special oil later on, but for now it is important to remember – *lavender is great for inducing a sense of calm*. Clary sage is another essential oil that has a particularly good effect in calming a patient's nerves. Derived from the steam distilled buds and leaves of the Clary Sage plant (*Salvea Sclarea),* this essential oil exhibits many parallel and complementary properties to lavender, especially when it comes to inducing a calmative effect. This remarkable herb has long been valued in its own right for its many and varied medicinal qualities, including its effect as an antidepressant, sedative and nervine agent. Care should be taken when using clary sage in combination with alcohol, as the herb can intensify the effects of this drug. Finally, geranium oil has been shown to be a highly effective emotional 'balancing' agent, which can greatly assist those suffering from anxiety or depression.

With the above calm inducing essential oils in mind, we'll now take a look at how to combine these into a great massage blend for stress relief. When making a blend for stress relief, it is perfectly acceptable to use a fairly neutral carrier oil, such as grapeseed as the primary constituent. This is because the essential oils are really doing the lion's share of the work here, and work in two distinct ways to create a feeling of calm. First, the scent of the essential oils works through the body's olfactory system to stimulate the limbic system, and helps to regulate impulses from the central nervous system that lead to an overactive adrenal response. For this reason, a carrier oil with a relatively neutral scent should be used here. The volatile compounds of the active essential oils also work by entering the body through the bloodstream; from here, they circulate throughout the body where they can relax muscles and also influence cortisol and adrenaline levels in the body by limiting overactive stress hormone production. As such, opting for a carrier oil with a moderately good rate of absorption (such as grapeseed or apricot kernel oils) is recommended.

With this in mind, the following treatment makes for a good remedy when treating stress in a patient: 3 drops of clary sage oil; 3 drops of lavender oil; 3 drops of geranium oil; 10mL grapeseed oil. All ingredients should be combined in a dark glass jar and shaken to combine. When applying via massage, the applicant should take a small amount of the blend (about the size of a dime) and rub together in their palms to warm before applying to the patient. Focus the massage on the back and shoulders, which can carry a lot of tension in a person experiencing high levels of stress. If you have more time, a full body massage can provide great benefits to a patient suffering from stress. Apply the same technique to the legs, arms, back, neck, shoulders, feet, hands and head. A comprehensive massage such as this (which can take around 45 minutes to an hour) can ensure the complete relaxation of the recipient as they become fully immersed in the experience. Good results can also be achieved using what is known as the *raindrop technique* which will be discussed further in the later chapter on meditation.

Find it by clicking here or type this link into your web browser: http://amzn.to/1C5NDCf

www.ingramcontent.com/pod-product-compliance
Lightning Source LLC
Chambersburg PA
CBHW070934290526
45795CB00003B/1012